THE
accidental
CÂRER

THE

accidental

CARER

A practical guide through uncertainty
by palliative home carers.

ROS CAPPER

First published 2017 by Reinventors NZ Ltd.

PO Box 32016. Devonport, Auckland 0744, New Zealand.

www.accidentalcarer.com

Edited by Janet McAllister and Dr Paul Vincent – www.doctoredit.co.nz
Designed by Victoria Wigzell – www.victoriawigzelldesign.co.nz
Printed by Benefitz – www.benefitz.co.nz

ISBN: 978-0-473-38303-9

To little Minna Capper,
who wholeheartedly loved her grandparents
through uncertain times.

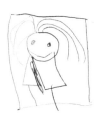

CONTENTS

Within palliative care, it remains rare to hear directly from the real experts in caring – the families and friends of the person diagnosed with an end of life illness. This book adds crucial new information from palliative home carers about what improved their caring experience.

Living with a life limiting illness is one of the hardest challenges we face as human beings. And the challenge is one shared by family, whānau, and friends. Our research has shown that they provide care and support with huge commitment and skill, but typically with little professional support.

The Accidental Carer is an important work. In it Ros shares her hard won knowledge and expertise of providing palliative care for her husband, Mike, with courage and humour. She also provides an avenue for other families to do the same. The gift she gives us in doing so is immeasurable.

If you are reading this guide because you are supporting someone with a life limiting illness, then I am convinced you will find the information it contains both invaluable and unique. I am not aware of a similar resource in New Zealand. If you are a reader with a professional interest in palliative care, I'm sure you will glean important new insights to help your work.

Ros is a remarkable woman. Most of us after going through a journey like hers would not have the energy or commitment to create a resource for the benefit of others. But she has, for which I am extremely grateful, as I am sure you will be too. It has truly been a privilege for our team to support her and this project.

Merryn

PROFESSOR MERRYN GOTT
Director, Te Arai Palliative Care and End of Life Research Group
University of Auckland

YOU MATTER

Warm Greetings.

The Accidental Carer – A Practical Guide Through Uncertainty by Palliative Home Carers is primarily for palliative carers who are caring for a family member diagnosed with an end-of-life illness. It is also for palliative carers' families and friends, and professional support people.

The Guide's purpose is to shine a light on practical choices made by palliative carers in their different situations in Aotearoa New Zealand. It has deliberately been kept brief for busy multi-tasking people!

I was a home-based palliative carer for my husband Mike for three years. Palliative care is care that gives comfort – it does not cure. During that time I noticed the lack of information written by home-based palliative carers about their hands-on experiences. In addition to my own reflections, this Guide includes contributions by four different family groups.

The website www.accidentalcarer.com has been designed to accompany this Guide and contains significant content not in the book including the experiences of other home-based palliative carers.

There are likely to be imperfections in this pioneering resource. Your feedback would be greatly appreciated to assist others embarking on this journey. Please send it to: ros@accidentalcarer.com.

Ros X

ROS CAPPER

Structure of this guide

There are important themes threaded throughout this Guide, such as the need to reach out for help, and to look after yourself as carer as well as the person you're caring for. The impact of uncertainty is 'coloured in' by carers living this common experience.

The Guide's structure loosely moves from practicalities to deeper issues. You do not need to read the sections in order.

Note: The focus of this Guide is on non-medical care, 'the glue that holds things together'. Skip what does not reflect your unique experience and adapt as you explore what could be useful to you.

1

INTRODUCTION

'You have drawn the short straw,' the Oncologist advised Mike and me. Mike's prostate cancer had spread, and he was advised his life was limited. We were shocked. As I paid for car parking while Mike sat in the car, I knew life had just shifted forever.

Supported by our 'Home Team' of friends, family and health professionals who generously gave their love, skills and other resources, I was Mike's palliative carer for three years while working part time. Mike was a gentle, gracious person who enjoyed thoughtful conversations, his family and opera.

Palliative care is care that gives comfort – it does not cure. If the person you are caring for has an illness with an uncertain future, you may be called a 'palliative carer' by those in the medical system. This Guide emerged from my exploring afterwards what I did not know at the time. The lack of information written by home-based palliative carers intrigued me. What I at first thought was a gap I soon realised was a chasm, hidden in plain sight.

So as far as I am aware, this Guide, designed to shine a light on the choices made by palliative carers at home, is the first of its kind in New Zealand. To everyone who reads this Guide, I genuinely hope it inspires you to do your best – that is all we as carers can do. Just as importantly, I hope it encourages you to reach out for help – palliative care is not something to do alone at home.

Sharing stories is an age-old way of making meaning, being inspired and strengthening our spirits to carry on. The stories of five family groups of home-based palliative carers (including my own) are here to support others as they embark on a journey of uncertainty, mystery, multi-tasking and unanticipated gifts.

How are you?
How are you really?

I've repeated this question in case you are used to answering 'Fine!' with a big smile, no matter what.

Sometimes when I was a palliative carer, I didn't want to talk about what was happening. I wasn't telling myself how I was. Other times it was a relief to share. When it comes to sharing, it is always your choice.

I am asking how you, the palliative carer, are today. Sometimes, I know, you may hear yourself answering with the medical details of the person you are caring for – because that has likely become your focus – and often the focus of the person asking the question.

I'm gently asking how you are in this situation … because how *you* are is important.

Caring for a very ill person at home is a 'big ask'

Tip: Wondering if you will 'cope' is normal.

Serious illness can come out of the blue. How many families are prepared for this? How many are prepared for the not knowing and what that may or may not mean? This is tough stuff.

Caring Choices Story: Taking it one day at a time

Anne* was diagnosed with an end-of-life illness. Her sister Diana writes of her experience as a palliative carer at Anne and her husband Robert's home:

At the beginning I was quite apprehensive, and really wondered if I would be able to take on a caring role with Anne. Illness had always frightened me. But I found that if I could focus on just one day, and even one step, at a time, and not get caught up with anxiety over the future, I could cope. I was amazed. As each new situation presented itself, I just met it, doing my best for Anne. It was all about her, moment by moment.

* Names have been changed.

Common next steps may include:
- grappling with what the facts may be – which takes time
- tests, scans, more tests and consultations
- managing the transport involved
- managing the car parking, costs included
- trying to absorb what the Specialist is saying
- driving home and going over both the said and the unsaid
- wondering what it all means
- wondering how to handle this new situation
- wondering what the new situation is exactly … begin the above again!

Caring Choices Story: Mystery

Pleasance, who cared for her partner Jane for the last three years of her life, writes:

Shortly after my partner Jane received her 'incurable' diagnosis, we heard that the Tibetan monks were in Auckland. So we went to watch them meditate and create an exquisite sand mandala. We knew that at the end, they'd ceremonially brush it all away, to signify the impermanence of life. It felt very poignant. I watched Jane watching the monks. She went very still and quiet ... she seemed completely absorbed in what they were doing. All I could do was stand beside her, equally quiet, wondering how it was for her. When they had brushed away the last vestiges, she turned to me, and said 'Let's go'. I felt I'd just witnessed someone bravely facing their death, and somehow taking strength from what the monks were doing. It seemed to be a turning point.

Our first family sharing time

Tip: Creating space for sharing, when you and your family feel ready, can help.

The week of Mike's diagnosis, our family had a heart-to-heart conversation over a shared lunch in a café. Our sons, Tim and Guy, and Mike and I all squeezed into a booth, ordered drinks and then looked at each other.

We'd got this far – now what? Mike's recent diagnosis meant we were all in shock.

Somehow, during that lunch we managed to acknowledge Mike's news and likely earlier-than-expected death, and our deep sadness. Tim and Guy began to recall special times with their Dad and the conversation literally climbed towards the times Mike went climbing with his young sons in the mountains. They shared how important these and other adventures with Mike were. And there were tears, silences, loving looks and hugs.

Our sons decided they would one day climb in the mountains together again. As we left, Tim said, 'Well, I've never had a conversation like that before!' Our shared lunch beautifully eased the way for later private one-to-one conversations.

Bringing friends and family 'into the loop' in a nourishing way

Tip: Having friends and family gather around can strengthen bonds for the way ahead.

Our friends and family pitched in to organise a surprise 'long table lunch' for Mike's birthday a month after his diagnosis. Friends cooked the food and hosted the lunch for us. Trisha generously offered her Waiheke retreat as the venue.

During the lunch people spontaneously rose to their feet one by one, sharing their love for Mike by warmly recalling special memories as our granddaughter and her small cousins cavorted over the couch. This experience was 'heart-warming family' at its best, drawing everyone into the circle of our new life situation early on. Mike clearly felt loved and we both felt well supported.

- Would getting together with people you choose be a good idea?
- Would one or more of them organise this with you?
- Would having a meal together be a good way to do this?

2

MANAGING
THE MEDICAL SIDE
OF THINGS

Medical appointments

Multiple medical appointments can mark the beginning of your changed life. Be gentle with yourself, as these situations will probably be new to you. The medical information about your ill family member may increase as you attend these appointments, and it is entirely possible that you won't remember all that was said at the previous one!

Information choices

- Do reach out for assistance with medical words.
- You and the ill person* can choose to meet with their General Practitioner (GP) or local Pharmacist for clarifying conversations about the illness and prescriptions (see below).
- You can ask a family member or friend for help to understand what you were both told. You can invite them to come with you to appointments too.
- As you are not the patient, either you go to appointments together with the ill person or you have their written permission to clarify information for them (you know how it is with privacy these days!)

* 'ill person' is used mainly in this Guide instead of 'patient' when referring to someone being cared for at home.

General Practitioners (GPs)

The ill person's GP can get to know you both and answer questions about the illness, the medicines, test results and how the health system works.

- They can refer their patient's details to the hospital-based Needs Assessment Service Coordination agency (NASC) who will then be in touch.
- There may be a mix of appointments between the Specialist at the hospital and the GP.
- All the reports from Specialists and tests go to the GP (or should do).
- The GP can be changed if their patient prefers this, especially when there is an uncertain diagnosis in the mix.

- An Oncologist is a specialist in cancer illnesses and can advise on the diagnosis and the likely outcome. The Radiologist can interpret things like MRI and CAT scans.

This is an awful lot of information to absorb. You may need a cup of tea and a lie down!

GP checklist

- The GP is seen as the Coordinator of Care when there is an end-of-life diagnosis.
- How comfortable is the ill person with their GP? Should a change of GP be considered?
- Do they see the same GP each time? Has the GP seen the ill person recently? When dealing with Specialists, keep the GP in the loop as to what is happening too.
- Will the GP visit at home if needed?
- Has the Specialist or GP arranged for NASC to assess the ill person for care support? This can take time, so do ask if it is happening (see Section 4 for more information on the support available).

Pharmacists

Tip: Ask your Pharmacist for help with medical information and medicines that are unfamiliar.

Our lovely local Pharmacists were happy to share with us how they support their palliative care customers. They were able to identify me as a palliative carer by the medications I was collecting for Mike, and by the questions I was asking.

Pharmacists can 'chunk' medical information into bite-sized pieces. Bite-sized information is easiest to digest. Carers trying to understand the illness and the medicines prescribed often ask Pharmacists for help. It costs nothing and you don't need an appointment.

I was appreciative of our Pharmacist Nichola's human touch – her look of compassion and her noticing if anything was not right with the prescription, putting us on her 'reminder list' to be called to see if repeats were needed.

Next is a list of the services your Pharmacist can provide. You may be surprised. I was!

Pharmacist services
Allan Pollock of Belmont Pharmacy, Auckland, contributed this list of services that Pharmacists can provide – just ask:

Pharmacists are the medicines experts you don't have to make an appointment to see. Pharmacists can:
- help translate 'medical gobbledygook' into plain English. Many customers have multiple and varied health providers, and we can cut through communication roadblocks to get timely information from them (we have the ability – with your permission – to look online at hospital notes to support this process).
- synchronise quantities so that different medicines run out at the same time and look at simplifying the sometimes complicated multiple drug, multiple dosing time regime.
- blister-pack all your medicines or prepare a medicines dosing chart explaining each drug's purpose and when to take it.
- deliver medicines to you at home (some pharmacies).

Managing medical information

Tip: Note things down in one place as your mind may not be!

Have you thought of putting all the medical papers in one place? Information to note in addition could include:
- advice that sounds useful
- comments you want to remember
- questions that come to you at 3am!
- the next appointment

Decide what works best for you:
- a notebook
- your phone
- the spaces in this Guide
- a folder with plastic sleeves

Choose one place – it saves time and removes the pressure of last-minute hunting!

Caring Choices Story: Medical treatment choices

Tane, who with his whānau (family) helped look after his Nan for the last five weeks of her life, says:

Nan made most decisions herself with guidance from the rest of us. The only tricky area was with chemo – whether to continue it or not when she didn't like how she felt after the first chemo treatment.
'It's up to you,' I advised her. 'You don't have to do it.'
'Don't I?' Nan replied.
'We're here to support you no matter what,' I said.
The next day she advised the medical people 'I don't want to (continue)'. It was quite an epiphany moment – you could see her feeling empowered.

Humour may sometimes be the best choice

Imagine you have managed to help your ill person into the car, driven on the busy motorway, and arrived at the small car park set aside for cancer patients near the Oncology Clinic at Auckland Hospital.

The car park is on a slope with a huge oak tree in the middle. At one end is a wire fence at the top of a steep cliff. You and other families are all driving an ill person around this space trying to score one of about 15 spaces. A competition for a park! You think this is a fantasy? No, that was my real situation in 2014. And as I circled I fantasised …

My fantasy was that we would be welcomed by a smiling valet who would park the car and that Mike would walk straight into the clinic leaning on a staff member's strong arm instead of walking with his stick up a slope. My outlandish fantasy helped me cope with the outlandish reality!

3

PRIORITIES
GUIDE DECISIONS

Priorities guide decisions

Tip: Clarify what is most important to you before making decisions.

When we first received Mike's diagnosis, these were my priorities:
- Mike would have the best care.
- I would continue my flexible part-time employment.
- Our four-year-old granddaughter Minna would usually stay overnight once a week. She brought us joy!

Later on, I added:
- I would sustain myself.

Having these priorities helped guide decision-making and encouraged me to ask for help.

Choosing my priorities early meant less to think through with each decision. For example, in relation to my first priority of 'Mike having the best care', it was important that Mike was able to make all his appointments on time. He needed to be driven and I prefer to drive outside peak traffic times. Mike therefore asked the appointment booking person for times that met these needs, and his appointments were arranged to suit. On some occasions, friends offered to drive Mike to help ensure no appointments were missed.

What are your important priorities right now?

My priorities are:

_____

_____

_____

_____

_____

Consider not doing everything that needs doing!
Tip: Share your growing to-do list.

Delegation is a wonderful thing at times like this. Please consider practising it!

Each person has their own list of 'everything that needs doing'. Mine for example included: driving to medical appointments, a part-time work position, hosting visitors, cooking, cleaning, attending to emails, important conversations with Mike, our sons and medical visitors – and always the laundry!

I could not do everything that needed doing by myself. Can you? In the end it comes down to a choice between:

- trying to do everything
 or
- deciding you cannot do everything and reaching out for help

If you decide not to try and do everything yourself, there are various decisions to be made (and revisited) to make sure priorities get done:

- Possibly the first choice will be who you can have a conversation with – a person who can listen well and assist you and the ill person to think through the options and preferences to meet both your priority needs. Who might this be?
- Which things will you ask for help with, and which things will you do yourself?
- Which things will you ask professionals to help with, and which things family and friends?

I learned to pace myself as best I could and change my mind as I experimented with things I could do myself, things I needed to ask for help with, and things that would no longer get done as regularly, if at all. I encourage you to try experimenting to find out what works best for you.

What is your life situation?

Does your life need to change or be totally rearranged now?
- What do you choose to keep doing because it is important to you? (Priorities!)
- What can you be flexible about?
- What do you need to be honest about? (can be just to yourself)
- What do you know you need help with?

Choices sometimes need to be changed

Tip: Feeling overwhelmed? Consider changing your choices.

Things change ... what works well today might not tomorrow. Arrangements are not set in concrete and can usually be changed to suit changing needs.

You may feel the need to:
- make choices that enable you to stay well
- ask for help to clarify your situation and consider choices that previously looked radical, for example taking a break while the ill person is temporarily cared for by others at home, or in the hospital or hospice (if the one near you offers this service)
- consider adding 'sustaining myself the best way I can' to your list of priorities

Some choices may feel bold because you have not made them before – well, you can be bold – or boldish! (if not now, when?).

Review your choices whenever you feel the need

Try reviewing your choices without self-judgement: 'It is how it is.'

Are you:
- comfortable in your role of palliative carer at the moment?
- comfortable-ish?
- feeling unsure about being in this role?
- needing hands-on assistance with anything?

- enjoying caring for your family member?
- feeling useful?
- wondering if you have made the right choice/what other choices there may be?
- all of the above at different times?(!)

Add anything not there that best suits your situation, for example:

- **I wonder what is the best way to**

_____

_____

_____

- **I wonder whether I can**

_____

_____

_____

- **I wonder whether I should**

_____

_____

_____

- **I wonder who would**

_____

_____

_____

What do you think needs to change or at least be tweaked? Note those things below, then ask for a conversation with a good listener to help you weigh the options. Reaching out in this way helps to attract your Home Team. People usually like to be asked for help.

The professional care option

Tip: You have choices.

If you are caring for someone at home with an end-of-life diagnosis it is good for you to know that help is 'out there'. It is a matter of accessing it, coordinating it, and sometimes paying for it.

Caring Choices Story: Seeking all available help

Pleasance, who cared for her partner Jane, writes:

Alongside the emotional and practical support we were receiving from our friends, we also sought out other care options to see what was available to us. The most successful 'intervention' was the woman who came in on a daily basis and showered Jane when she couldn't do it any longer. She was very good at it, in a matter-of-fact way, and Jane ended up looking and feeling refreshed, ready for whatever the day might bring – a cup of coffee with me down in Ponsonby Road, a visit, whatever it was that we had planned.

Exploring professional care

You may be able to get free or subsidised professional help with:

- 'personal cares'
    - showering, or washing in bed
    - meal preparation
    - medicine prompting
    - toileting
    - regular linen changes
    - special bed equipment
- housework (if you have a Community Services card)
- shopping support (if you have a Community Services card)

Check access to these by having a conversation about carer choices with your GP and/or the hospital-based Needs Assessment Service Coordination agency (NASC) to help you and the person you care for make a decision that works for both of you.

NASC is very important for palliative care. Your GP, Specialist, and other health professionals can refer ill people to NASC and may already have done so for the person you care for. NASC provides access to various 'cares' depending on the assessment of needs. If the ill person is assessed as needing 'personal cares', NASC will contact a care agency who will visit you both at home to assess who may be best to assist the ill person. NASC will also contact the District Nurse if a wound needs attending or special equipment such as an electric bed or commode needs to be delivered to your home.

There are also private care providers you can use. Enquire at your GP consulting rooms or local Age Concern or Citizens Advice Bureau for information – or ask a member of your Home Team (see Section 5) to do this for you.

Your local hospice can help you and the ill person access services. Hospice community nurses can visit people at home to assess and advise on services available. While they do not provide personal cares as a rule, they can help you to access resources. For example, they may suggest care in hospice for the ill person for a week while your home is readied for home care or to give you a break, or to sort out the medicines being used. This will depend on the hospice assessment of the ill person and the availability of accommodation.

Carer choices around physical care

Tip: You never know how well something may turn out!

I made the choice to not usually provide physical care myself, such as personal washing.

It was Christmas. The Oncologist sent our details to NASC. NASC contacted a care agency to provide Mike's physical cares and they came to our home to interview us. The wonderful Rachel came twice a day, six days a week to wash Mike and make his bed. 'Let's just make do on Sundays,' requested Mike. And so we did.

Rachel was from China. Mike was so happy to feel useful by teaching her everyday English. Rachel's visits raised his morale and gave me more choices on how I used my time. We arranged for the paper edition of the daily newspaper to be delivered so that Mike and Rachel could look at the news stories together and have conversations.

Each morning when Rachel arrived, I had an hour to go to the supermarket or walk, or meet a friend in a café. One day, two happy faces greeted me. 'Go on,' said Mike to Rachel, 'tell Ros what you learned!' Rachel advised me with a smile: 'It is not ... the end ... of the world!'

They were both so proud of their achievements: Mike enjoyed contributing to Rachel's language needs and Rachel loved learning everyday phrases she could use. How cool is that?

I was grateful this arrangement worked so well for us all over five key months.

4

HOW A HOME-CARE HOME MAY BE DIFFERENT

How are you going so far? Absorbing the medical information is one thing, but wondering what it all means and focusing on one step at a time can be another.

Palliative carers: You matter! Please bring your needs into the picture as routines change – heck, life is changing all the time. Uncertainty and grief may be showing up.

Try to keep your top priorities in mind as you make decisions in consultation with others involved. The experiences of palliative caring at home by five families is key to the information in this Guide: five families doing what families have done through the ages – caring for an ill family member in their own home, giving comfort care to the best of their ability while keeping a watchful eye for when more will be needed at times.

Examples of where more help might be needed include:
- lifting a heavy ill person
- showering
- assessment or review of the situation with the ill person and the carer(s)
- organising respite from intense caring
- advice on mobility and equipment for that

This is not about 'fixing things' or a cure. Rather, palliative home care can ease the way for an ill person to make the most of how things are and choose their priorities, if time is short. It can also ease the way for family members to engage with each other and the ill person about things that matter to them. Younger family members will watch how older people manage this situation, which is how family traditions are built.

Everyone involved is facing uncertainty. A phone call from a relation living overseas asking when they should book their flight to see the ill person can have the family at home practically gibbering in uncertainty. Put simply, no one really knows for sure.

Family members who are competent planners, managers and organisers in their daily lives can find these skills redundant in this situation of 'not knowing' and learn new skills of living in the moment.

The daily routine

An ex-palliative carer confided: 'I needed the day's routine laid out for me on paper. I had no nursing background and it's different from looking after small children. I'm used to teaching people how to do parts of my professional job. No one did this for me in this situation.'

In response to this plea, here are some ideas to consider while pacing yourself one step at a time and experimenting in your unique situation:

- Needs vary from person to person and household to household so 'pick and mix' from ideas and choices in this Guide and from what you are learning on the job.
- Wanting a routine is understandable if you're unused to illness and trying to manage a household. So let's help: firstly, if the ill person is mainly bedbound, their care needs to first be assessed by their GP.
- You as the palliative carer are the best person to decide what you wish to be responsible for and what you prefer to not do as you consider your needs and choices. You do *not* have to do *everything* on your own. You will need to advise your GP and/or Needs Assessors of your preferences after you have had a conversation with the ill person and possibly other family members.
- You can ask a friend or family member or agency carer to share care on a regular basis to ensure you have the necessary opportunity for time alone to B R E A T H E, walk outside, stock up on supplies and/or meet a friend if you want to.
- On a day-to-day basis, be guided by how the ill person is and respond when they're hungry, thirsty or need to move while responding to your own needs too.

The suggestions on these pages will vary with each person – take note of what you see and hear and what your instinct tells you. Ask for help when unsure.

Here are some loose guidelines to try out (if there's one certainty it is that these will change!):

Early morning: Check first thing how the ill person is, what sort of night they had and if they need pain relief and/or nausea control. Keep notes of medications taken if the ill person is not doing that. Some people manage their own medications and some need help. Early morning can be a good time for a chat. Morning talks can be deeply important to a person who has been awake reflecting (you and them!).

Personal comfort: Do they need changing/assistance with toileting? If a carer is coming in, bed changes and washing would be undertaken by them.

Food and drinks: Generally offer food/drinks at appropriate meal times if the ill person is eating. However, keep in mind that some people eventually refuse food/drinks. Don't be concerned if everything offered is not finished. Very small portions may be preferred. Appetites can change.

Washing: After breakfast, if the ill person is mainly in bed, having a wash in bed assists basic hygiene and comfort. Special cream for their back may be prescribed. A plastic washing up bowl, soap, flannel and towel are all that is needed. If you are uncomfortable or need help, be sure to tell the GP or NASC so that arrangements can be changed. You can share with others to clarify your thinking.

A 'walker' to go to the toilet is helpful for those who need to balance themselves as they walk. Equipment may be accessed through NASC or District Nurses and will be delivered. For suppliers of continence products, including online ones, see www.accidentalcarer.com

Entertainment: Reading, music, TV, audio books, being read to, headphones and/or portable devices are enjoyed by many. Silence is preferred by some. Conversations may enable you to know what is most wanted – just ask!

Visitors: Some people welcome all visitors who come while others prefer very few or none. If visitors are welcome, just advise family and friends of time preferences. You can ask them to text or call ahead about the best time and, if you and the person you are caring for need a daily nap, timetable that in first to provide needed rest. Some visitors are not comfortable around illness and may be best hosted with a drink in the lounge first! Home Team members can attend to this when you have other priorities.

Settling at night: This can be helped by a face-and-hands wash and teeth cleaning and a chat. Place a bell within reach of the ill person for help if bedbound. Note down medications taken. A Thermos of their favourite warm drink and 'bendy' straws can be a comfort during the night, placed within reach. A child's sipper cup or bendy straw works well for cold drinks (lying in bed can make drinking from cups tricky). Night lights and a torch can help prevent falls.

A typical day's routine

Note: Things change constantly. This was how it was at that time.

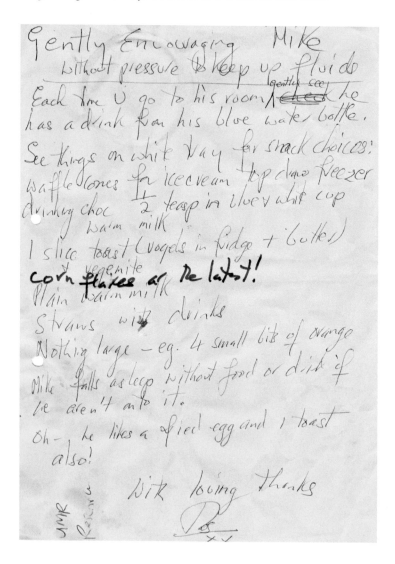

A typical day's routine, sketched in my (rough!) writing, for family members taking over care for two nights and days.

Mike and I fell in love again!

Five in the morning became our main sharing time. We'd reminisce as the birds sang the new day in. I sat close to Mike as we shared our peak life experiences amidst busy international lives with children. It was very emotional, and brought our love full centre. Past challenging times were now as shadows as we reminisced about such experiences as:

- walking for hours in the snow in Czechoslovakia carrying skis
- dragging a pine tree through the snow in London and standing it on the Hampstead carpet, inviting friends to come see our beautiful snow-covered Christmas tree – they opened the door to a tree sitting in a puddle of water on the posh carpet, bringing laughter at this basic physics stuff-up!
- living in a motor home in London, driving off each morning in a hurry with dishes sliding to get Tim to school on time
- skiing trips to Mt Ruapehu with friends, sharing a house, snow adventures, meal cooking and sparkly conversations over wine

These sharing times, we reflected, were the 'glue experiences' that had everyone pitching in naturally again now – we can do this! Past adventures brought joy as we coloured in our memories. How lucky were we to have this time to do this now!

Arranging your home as a home-care home

Care bedroom

Home care takes up home space. You may need a friend's garage to store stuff, as we did! The main thing is how much room a hospital-type bed can take up.

Decluttering is important to have space to move around the bed and enable trays to be positioned for easy access from the bed. Our sons spent a weekend removing everything that would not be needed from the bedroom.
We kept in the room things that were familiar: favourite pictures, the laptop, radio, mobile phone, landline phone and torch, and added fresh flowers and

music when desired. We made do with a collapsible chair for visitors until we cleared more space!

Electric beds are 'bony' metal single-bed constructions that gently move and usefully enable the ill person's back to stay in good condition. It is impossible for two people to lie comfortably together in an electric bed. We grew to hate the bed, while appreciating that it was keeping Mike's back in good shape.

A tip for health professionals
For anyone in a relationship, it would be good to know ahead of time that their embracing in bed together is about to end. When a person is at their most vulnerable, the familiar comfort of an embrace is withdrawn. A palliative carer confided 'the electric bed broke the connection, our closeness'. A 'heads up' two days beforehand would have been greatly appreciated by the couple.

Home-care kitchen
With people in our Home Team regularly visiting, I found making the most commonly enjoyed drinks easier by placing a large white plastic tray on the kitchen bench loaded with the necessities. No one needed to hunt them down or put them in unlikely(!) places afterwards. The white tray eased the way for us all to participate in Mike's care – you'd hear 'Look on the white tray!' as someone searched for the Horlicks to make Fortisip more appetising.

The tasting plate
When Mike's appetite became so small it hardly earned the name, I created a 'tasting plate' with a variety of 'small somethings' for him to choose from. I chose our very best flowery German porcelain platter-of-happy-memories and placed on it wee spoons of the 'tastes' Mike now preferred, using inexpensive china spoons for easy eating.

Choices varied depending on daily preferences. They could include spoons of (hot) baked beans, peeled pear, peeled kiwifruit or finger toast or scrambled egg.

I would leave the room for a bit so as Mike could taste his choices without feeling watched and judged!

I enjoyed seeing my favourite plate from long ago dinner parties being used again. In fact all of the above could have been more for me than Mike! Well, that's OK too.

If the person you are caring for is eating little and therefore losing weight, this can be very uncomfortable for a carer who is doing their best. It is human nature to want someone to 'eat up' – but not always appropriate.

Be guided by the ill person, and if concerned, chat about contacting their GP.

Foods that had previously been enjoyed may no longer appeal – nor favourite drinks. That is how it is with some illnesses.

The costs of caring at home

Tip to friends and family: The main carer may welcome a money chat.

Being a palliative carer is expensive. Being a working carer whose job hours need to be shortened or abandoned altogether creates real financial pressure. Car parking charges at the hospitals mount up. Petrol does too, especially when attending appointments nowhere near your home.

Cleaning is often not available free and some people pay for the extra cleaning needed in a home-care home. Many buy special foods the ill person might enjoy, which are often expensive. There may be costly cultural food expectations to live up to. In our case, the unanticipated cost of the St John Ambulance for a 10 minute ride to hospice was $200. Who knew?

If you are wondering how you will manage financially, and costs are straining your budget, be sure to seek help, and accept it if offered. The ill person may be eligible for financial support through Work and Income if they have needed to leave their employment. Initiate this process early – there is no 'back pay'!

Where to find advice on financial assistance:
- the Work and Income website (www.workandincome.govt.nz) gives you the basics of available support. (If negotiating a complex website is in the 'too-hard basket', ask a friend or family member to do this on your behalf.)
- the hospice social workers, if the person you are caring for is registered with the local hospice
- your local Work and Income office
- the Needs Assessment Service Coordination agency (NASC)

Accepting offers of financial help can ease the way and lower your anxiety.

The use of crowdfunding sites such as Givealittle (www.givealittle.co.nz) in illness situations is common. Your Home Team (see Section 5) may like to assist with this.

The thought Police
Tip: There are no such people but we can easily imagine there are!

Ha ha! If you are a palliative carer doing your best in a new situation, of course you'll find yourself wondering if what you're doing is 'right' and whether you'll be criticised for your choices. Imagining people will judge your choices is common and anxiety-causing. You may be feeling the most vulnerable you ever have. Try showing yourself the same depth of compassion you would with a dear friend.

You will be doing your best *and* asking for help and advice, won't you? My wise friend Julie Diamond used to ask: 'May I give you some unasked-for advice?' Whoever asks beforehand? – her question always made me laugh.

Caring Choices Story: Uncertainty

Jackie's husband Kevin had been given an end-of-life diagnosis and had recently responded well to immunotherapy. Jackie recalls how tough she found things a year before his improvement:

'A year or so ago when he was at his worst, I feel I really didn't cope at all well, and would burst into tears frequently, both at home and often to complete strangers. I would feel guilty that I was so upset, when it wasn't even me going through the nightmare. North Shore Hospice's counsellor was a wonderful help in this regard, as was meeting up with other carers in the same position.'

Caring Choices Story: Support through uncertainty

Pleasance, who cared for her partner Jane, writes:

There was the terror sitting and waiting for me, when I went to bed each night. But if that's how I felt, how much worse must it be for her? We used audio recordings* by Beverley Silvester-Clark for people facing terminal illness: one for 'last thing at night', another one for the morning, and a third that would come in very handy when Jane began her chemo treatment. The atmosphere in our home began to change. Friends noticed it, coming in. It was like there were 'other presences' with us, accompanying us on this tough journey. Friends also took notice because it was Jane – not me, the one usually associated with more 'way out there' practices, and beliefs. No, this was Jane – known for having her feet firmly on the ground, and fond of saying she 'had a bob both ways' in terms of medical intervention and the more spiritual side. So as our home atmosphere softened; somehow these recordings gave me strength too.

* Visit www.accidentalcarer.com for details of these recordings.

Perfection is not required!

Tip: Try believing this because the alternative causes anxiety!

An ex-palliative carer confides: 'I still feel guilty I didn't do a good job. They said I did but I didn't.'

Most palliative carers will feel anxious at some point. It's unlikely that you or others will be perfect throughout this experience. There will be times when things go 'pear-shaped'. Expect this. And yes, things going pear-shaped is very hard to experience when you're doing your best.

With appointments, new information, and probably a 'to do' list coming out of your ears, you can find yourself trying to 'get things right' and getting into a tizz as a result. This is entirely understandable. You will do your best and try your hardest, however everything will not be perfectly done as agreed: not at home, hospital or with family. People are not perfect. There are likely to be mismatches of expectations.

When I was feeling most pressured and keen for things to go well for Mike, and an expected thing did not happen, my options were:

- drop my expectations
- ask for change
- get into a tizz (sometimes I did not do this with grace – good luck!)

5

THE HOME TEAM
AND CARING CHOICES

The choice to attract and grow your home team
Tip: 'Open a door' for others to come alongside you.

Medical professionals are advisory. A Home Team can be the loving 'glue' that keeps things – and you! – together.

When Mike was unexpectedly admitted to hospital, and I had a work commitment, a friend drove across Auckland to be with him – unasked. Wow! Christina's initiative gave me an important clue: I don't need to do everything myself.

In time, friends and family and volunteers from organisations can become a welcome Home Team of drivers, loving companions, problem solvers, listeners and meal contributors. It is called 'Community' – the rewards of which are mutual, we were constantly told.

A wide variety of loving help followed news of our Mike's diagnosis:
- Barbara brought a tri-pillow to support Mike to sit more comfortably.
- Margaret brought her quality listening for 'conversations about things that matter'.
- Jan brought books on opera which Mike enjoyed.
- Guy brought humour, errand-going energy, and fun.
- Tim gave gentle encouragement and enabled Mike to access films in bed.
- Elisabeth drove Mike to medical appointments, staying with him.
- Sanna came with our grandchildren, who gave joy and cuddles.
- Trisha offered her retreat venue for our friends and family gathering.

Gratitude and good memories were the all-important outcomes for me.
- Would a family member or friend assist with specific tasks (e.g. driving)?
- Would you invite the most likely person or people for a tea or coffee to chat about this, or choose someone to ask others on your behalf?

If you are used to being independent, this may be unfamiliar and even seem unnecessary. I am just checking here whether you are edging towards asking for help but feeling uncomfortable, and you're going in a bit of a circle. Remember that the ill family member may take comfort from your having help.

There are a number of 'sharing tasks' apps available which your Home Team can use to keep everyone up to date and to stay in touch. There are apps designed specifically for coordinating in caring situations. Visit www.accidentalcarer.com for more details.

Caring Choices Story: A live-in home team

Tane, who helped look after his Nan during the last five weeks of her life, writes:

'Nan used to call me her 'Sunshine Boy' and she was my number one priority. She and Papa brought me up. I lived with them, my mother and cousins in a house next to the marae.

My Mum and five first cousins all gathered in the same house to care for Nan, with the cousins taking turns. The experienced hospice nurses knew our family and visited daily, picking up how we were managing and supporting that.

I felt lucky and grateful to be with her when she was dying and for nothing else to matter but her welfare …

Coming together as a family is just what we've always done, everyone coming together and making it work – usually it's Christmas and birthdays. My Grandfather used to say: 'God first, neighbours second and yourself last.'

Nan was a typical matriarchal figure – an amazing cook and baker who dedicated her life to the care and love of her family. Now everyone came to her. Some days she didn't want to see anyone.

EMBRACE
THE OPPORTUNITY
TO LOVE

We would put up a blackboard saying 'Hello, welcome, you're welcome to come in for a cup of tea but Nan isn't up to seeing anyone today.'

People kept coming with food and fruit and flowers – occasionally, if Nan was up to it, the person she used to have a wine with would join her in that!

She was Queen to a lot of people.

My tip for others: I'd give as much time as you can. Embrace the opportunity to love more than you ever thought possible. Nan spent her life giving love to others and it was amazing to see the love reciprocated in her last days. It was a wonderful example of karma.'

When people say 'just call if there's anything I can do'
Tip: Let's make this work for you!

Think who you could have a chat with about your new situation. Regular Home Team people appreciated their involvement, gained deeper friendships and good conversations, explored life questions new to them, and learned about gas stoves! 'I have never been in this situation,' said a friend who became a regular Home Team member.

- Receiving a diagnosis of a limited life is a common experience 'out there for others' but may be new to you and those close to you, as well as the person diagnosed.
- Intentionally growing a Home Team may seem a foreign concept, but as Tane advises, it is how things have always been for some family groups, whānau and cultures.
- When families are scattered far and wide there's the need to reach out and create your 'family' of friends, neighbours and professional support people. You may be surprised in a good way at who is attracted to join in.

Time to gather what's left of your wits!

- Who could you ask to have a cuppa with you for a Home Team conversation?
- Is there a friend you can ask to invite potential Home Team people to meet with you? (The friend may offer to host this.)
- Who can you or your friend phone or email or Facebook about it?
- You may welcome more 'thinking out loud' conversations as you live this experience. Who would be your best companion for these?

Caring Choices Story: 'The Clan'

Pleasance, who cared for her partner Jane, writes:

'One of the things Jane and I realised shortly after her diagnosis was that we needed to call on as much support as possible, from what we called 'The Clan' (our lesbian community). Jane was facing her death, and I had to face the fact that I was going to lose her, my life partner, lover and best friend for 25 years. It felt enormous. We knew we had to reach out.

We set about letting our closest friends know, and braced ourselves to deal with their horror and disbelief. Our friends in Wellington, where we'd lived together for almost 20 years of our lives, began travel plans immediately.

We also had close connections with friends in Auckland, who instantly asked what they could do to help. 'Come around and drink G&T's [gin and tonic] with P' was Jane's answer. Mine was a bit more practical. I explained to friends that while I'd be good at the emotional support side for Jane, the part that would 'go out the window' at this time of stress would be cooking. They understood.

So, we began a twice-weekly G&T session at our home with close friends, which fortunately included a couple of very good cooks! Other friends in the city began dropping off meals too when they visited, which lifted our spirits and kept us focused on what mattered: the quality of Jane's life, for whatever remained of it. It meant I could concentrate on what I was good at, rather than stressing about what I couldn't do. We also realised it really helped to have something specific to say, when friends asked how they could support us. The 'shock' of the diagnosis had moved us far beyond worrying about what other people would think. All we knew was that we were at a point where we had to be completely real.

The practical offers of help continued – e.g. one friend came and rearranged our linen cupboard; another one made chicken stocks and stacked them in the freezer. Often it was the gesture that counted, as much as the act itself.

One of the outstanding 'gifts' I take from that time was that I was not alone. I only had to ask.'

Caring Choices Story: Who should take charge?

Anne was ill and her husband Robert, sister Diana and daughter Karen planned to care for her at home with the support of the local nursing agency over several weeks. Taking cues from Anne helped decide the 'lead carer' and provided answers to the questions 'Who's taking charge?' and 'Who makes decisions?'

Diana writes:

'With several close family members involved in Anne's care during the last months of a short illness, I struggled with acknowledging who was in charge. Anne had recently married her partner of 10 years and I thought at times that he was bossy and taking control. 'Who does he think he is?' I thought. 'I'm the closest!' Sometimes we disagreed about treatment options or how to best help her.

By observing Anne I could see that the person she responded to most was her husband. This made it easier for me to step back and allow him to assume leadership, while openly discussing my opinions, hopes and fears. Having a lead carer worked well for us right through to the end. I can now see that it was entirely natural for him to take a lead … he loved her unconditionally, and she him. What I had reacted to as 'bossiness' was in fact practical and protective support of his partner. Their bond in no way threatened the close links and love Anne and I had shared as sisters for her entire lifetime. It was a team approach – we all worked together to give Anne the best care we could while running a household.'

Robert writes:

'It was very clear to me from the start that I was the one caring for Anne, with other family members helping out. Anne had been my partner and wife for nearly ten years; she was mine. But, of course, she also 'belonged' to others – close family who had known her far longer than I had – and they rightly felt similarly about their role as carers. Anne's sister had known her from birth; her daughter had known Anne for ever – who was this interloper?

And yet, just as I felt a little tension beginning to show, Anne's daughter made a very short, quiet statement: 'Anne is part of our lives by family connection, but she chose Robert to be her partner.'

The tension vanished, each of us accepting our part, our connection with Anne. It allowed me to assume a significant role without feeling as though I was a stranger who had just joined the party.

There was no conscious discussion about who would make particular decisions, no vote, no roundtable consensus – they seemed to happen naturally as Anne's sister and daughter graciously gave me just a little more space, or sought my views on what we might do next. Later on, when it seemed that more medication might be needed, or the bed needed to be changed, it felt OK for me to initiate it; in some ways I think that may have made it easier for the rest of the family to be able to be there supporting Anne, rather than having to think about what might be needed next.'

6

CREATIVE GIFTS

Creative gifts

Tip: Welcome friends and family being creative with their gifts.

Gifting choices

Useful gifting choices for the person caring for someone at home:

- Practical choices depend on the situation in that home.
- Is the ill person eating little and the palliative carer's social life limited? (their 'social life' may have shrunk to receptionists in waiting rooms).
- How involved would you consider being?
- Have you had a conversation with the carer about how she or he is, and offered a way you would like to contribute?
- Have you actioned your offer?

Having people check in, offer and action is a wonderful thing!

Gifting can meet both physical and social needs

Mike was eating little. I was drawn to toast some evenings! A friend gifted My Food Bag®. Two tall sturdy bags arrived with fresh vegetables in one and chilled meats, cheeses and sauces in the other, accompanied by recipes for four meals.

I was taken aback by the exotic-looking meal as I scanned a recipe for roast duck! 'Whaaaat!' I thought. But then an idea came to me: Invite a friend!

I texted Barbara, inviting her for dinner on a night she chose. The catch: she would cook it! I didn't have to shop or plan or think. Barbara was thrilled to be invited to this new experience. The duck, her companionship and the glass of wine were all very welcome.

What a fantastic way to have company, dinner and a catch up on gossip when your social life has shrunk! I'd just chop something Barbara gave me to chop up as we nattered. She did the actual cooking. Mike was happy knowing I was happy – and well fed.

Gradually I returned to the enjoyment of cooking and company and 'proper food'. The gifting was fortnightly. Different people shared the gifting and the eating. Thank you all!

Creative gift ideas

- Driving the ill person to some appointments (e.g. once a month). Carers: If the offer is by someone who can safely drive, park and accompany the ill person to their appointment, please accept, especially for a non-Specialist consultation.
- Your company some evenings, arriving with food and gossip! Check first, and judge how long to stay (e.g. between 10 minutes and an hour).
- A 'tower' shape of $20 of coins for car parking wrapped in pretty paper.
- Gardening – either for or with the person caring.
- A massage voucher linked to you staying with the ill person (if that is necessary) while the palliative carer has a massage (the ill person may like one too!)
- A pot plant or a plant from your garden.
- An offer to listen if the carer would like to confidentially discuss a thought or question with you.
- Start a campaign on a crowdfunding site such as Givealittle (www.givealittle.co.nz)
- Time. You can offer this in a card, being specific (e.g. 'I have the next three Thursdays free from 1–4pm to stay with X. Would this be useful? Please text or call if suits, love Tigger'). Carers: If you and the ill person are comfortable having this person stay for that time, you can attend to other priorities.
- A regular glass of wine together at a time that suits the carer.
- Regular G&T sessions – like The Clan's!

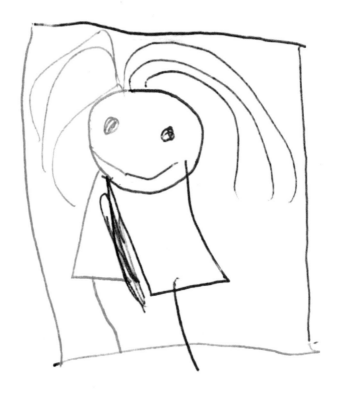

Minna. Self portrait.

To friends and family: the gift of caring for the carer

Tip: This may be a new situation for the main carer.

Your friend or family member may be anxious, shocked, experiencing grief, and not sleeping well. They may need you to be patient as they slowly make their way through this new situation. Have you asked them: 'How's it going for you?' Most people naturally ask about the ill person. The main carer may appreciate your asking how they are – not in front of the ill person though!

Your ability to not say anything if you think they are doing things 'wrong' or are irritable is an especially welcome gift! Their choices may be different from how you would do things – but it is unlikely to be life-threatening. They may be feeling exhausted and sensitive about how things are in their house.

The really good thing is to recognise that, well, it is all about love. Things that once seemed so important may no longer be so; it is quite radical as an experience, to have your priorities so swiftly rearranged.

To visitors: gift your listening to the carer's story

After you ask the carer 'How's it going?' or 'How are you?', try doing your best to focus on their reply and their situation. May I gently suggest you ask how your friend is doing and leave out comments like 'When I was looking after Doug …', even if this thought immediately springs to mind, and the situations seem similar.

However, do bring your whole self: your caring, love and the humour your friends and family enjoy about you – a bit of a juggle but you can do it!

The gift of living in the moment

Our four-year-old granddaughter Minna lived in the moment, as four year olds do, and clearly thought life was to be enjoyed – memories of yesterday or worries about the future were not for her. Life is Now! Even when I was tired, Minna being a regular guest was a priority. She brought joy and her style of

HOW'S IT GOING
FOR YOU?

beaming love encouraged us to live moment by moment, which was so helpful.

We created stories, had cuddles, laughed at jokes, shaped playdough, and lit candles to blow out loudly. What a nourishing way to be in life. She joyfully jumped from the sofa onto a cushion on the floor with happy shrieks of laughter. During my experience as a palliative carer, whenever I began thinking about the future or past when Minna was around, I was likely to be interrupted with a 'knock-knock' joke! – perfect for learning to live in the moment.

Palliative carers advise that helpful ways to support living in the moment include:
- being creative (e.g. enjoying a craft, especially one involving colours)
- meditation
- nature (the garden)
- favourite music

What or who is showing up in your life that may support you to live in the moment as best you can in a time of uncertainty?

Gifting happy memories

I contacted three men who had been friends of Mike's since the '80s and usually met as a group. I sensed this would be a good time for these special friends to have a private lunch with Mike.

His friends enthusiastically agreed and flew an hour north. I prepared lunch and left while these old friends enjoyed two hours of loving conversation. Their faces on my return were pure happiness, and remain a favourite 'happy memory' for me. Others learned of this lunch, and the pleasure spread.

The gift of instinct – the naughty bit (not asking permission)

Mike was keen to float in warm water when he was receiving chemotherapy. His Oncologist warned us about using public pools because of the risk of infection with a lowered immune system. If anything, this made Mike's desire for a pool float even greater. He knew his life was limited, so 'If not now, when?' was his driving thought.

We decided to be naughty – a thrill in itself! He floated in the heated public outdoor pool on a sunny day, aided by his plastic neck brace. Few people were around. Minna was with him, tickling his toes. I held towels, our car close by.

He enjoyed this twice – the float and the unusual feeling of being naughty. His beaming face said it all. If this was risk-taking, it was a risk he wanted to take.

7

THE CHOICE TO
SUSTAIN YOURSELF

The choice to sustain yourself

Tip: You may need to make further changes to prevent becoming overwhelmed.

Remember when you're on a plane and the cabin crew advise that if oxygen masks come down, you are to put yours on first before you attend to others? The reason is that if you do not access oxygen yourself, you will not have the capability to assist anyone else.

The same principle applies here: you and your health are very important.

If you are caring through uncertainty for a period of time, your health and spirit may gradually become affected – so gradually that you may not notice at first. Sometimes the ill person can become irritable, grumpy and unhelpful, which is hard. Sometimes you're heading that way yourself!

Please let people know what is going on for you both, what you need, and what you think might help – even if you can only squeak it out! Others cannot read your mind and may not know what is happening. I know sometimes it's hard to disclose you're not on top of things when you're used to 'getting things right' – however, the reality for most of us is that we're at times struggling with too much on too many levels

People to share with – to gain more support and creative options – include a friend, family member, hospice counsellor, Home Team member, GP, Needs Assessment Service Coordination agency (NASC) or a friend of the ill person. Online conversations with a trusted friend can be nourishing and supportive too.

Having someone else – or two people – take your place for two nights and days can be a way to clear your mind enough to review your situation.

Need a break from caring?

If the ill person is known by NASC, you can ask them about a carer temporarily taking your place. You can also ask about 'respite care' from the professional support people involved including your GP and hospice community nurse. This means the ill person will be cared for elsewhere for a few days. Alternatively, your Home Team family may wish to support you by taking your place for a couple of nights.

Is the number of visitors becoming overwhelming?
- Limit 'drop-in' visits by advising by text, email or phone that from X to Y time each day you and the ill person will be having a nap, or delegate this task to a member of your Home Team.
- Advise which times are best for visitors to come so that you can do errands/enjoy their company.
- Use Tane's blackboard idea (see Section 5).
- Hear offers made by people you are in conversation with instead of automatically dismissing them.

Needs and choices change. Experiment and check in with the person you are caring for.

If you know your energy is low and you need help to do any of the above, please ask for it.

Reviewing your situation as a Palliative Carer

Tip: What are you, the palliative carer at home, now seeing, feeling and sensing?

I have not read anywhere about what I am to write. Should I write this? (Thought Police!).

At first I was totally focused on the situation we began together: Mike's illness. We were a couple at medical appointments.

After a while – I'm not sure how long – I realised the medical path was not my personal path. I began to look for a door marked 'CARERS THIS WAY'! I was a beloved companion, but realistically we were on different future paths.

Mike's life would be shortened we were advised, and I could sense that. I acknowledged to myself that I would live beyond Mike. It was an honest, deeply sad and lonely realisation during our joint and energetic focus together on Mike's illness and his care.

I began to mentally prepare myself for what was likely to happen next. This was DIY. I struggled as I focused on Mike's increasing needs while living the gap in our futures.

This is so obvious looking back. My situation was unexplored in the medical appointments we kept. And there was no door marked 'CARERS THIS WAY'.

Self-comfort care
Tip: Take yourself seriously!

If you are 'losing the plot' in various ways or think you might be, check out the following choices other palliative carers have made when they have found themselves in tears, forgetting their passwords at the bank or feeling furious, their voice breaking with stress at the uncertainty of life. These are real, normal responses when you are exhausted, see no end in sight – and possibly feel guilty for thinking whatever you are thinking!

- Inviting a family member to stay (e.g. a sister).
- Asking for respite care for the ill person to give both people a break.
- Joining a hospice 'support group for palliative carers'.
- Gardening (can be rearranging pot plants or fierce digging!).
- Checking in with a good counsellor.
- Everyone fishing in a favourite spot with many family members in support.

- Swapping caring duties with someone for two nights to B R E A T H E and rediscover your instinct ... more than one of the above at once!

How can you best nourish yourself in a pressured situation?

Reaching out for a safe place where raw emotion is OK can be a good choice,

- are your feelings bubbling up once the practical tasks are more in hand?
- are you having a useful conversation about how you are feeling with anyone?
- would it be a good idea to arrange a time with a counsellor through Hospice or other services? (you don't have to have an agends – just a wish to talk about how things are for you).

Caring Choices Story: Taking breaks from intensive caring

Robert, who cared for his wife Anne, writes:

I found the intensive nature of caring for Anne to be both rewarding and tiring. I needed a break every couple of hours just to rebalance my energy, to move, and connect with the broader world for a few minutes, so that I could return and focus energy back into Anne. Sometimes it was the practical things such as bringing in some firewood that gave me a chance to appreciate that the world was continuing to turn; it also gave other family members the chance to be with Anne and confirm their own special bond with her.

Does it really matter?
Tip: Choosing your top priorities is key to self-care.

Asking 'does it really matter?' about anything even slightly complicated can bring lightness and laughter at ourselves for being ridiculous! Life is so precious and it can be a pleasure to let some things go and learn about not being perfect.

When someone is advised their life is likely limited and the palliative carer has limited time and energy to make everything matter, choose what really matters!

Examples of things that don't really matter:
* answering phone calls – create an answering message thanking people for their call and requesting them to please leave a message.
* matching anything – plates etc. – anything goes
* staying in touch with everyone you said you would – delegate instead
* keeping every agreement, especially when you're not up to much – hang loose!
* making top-notch meals – try buying in or being a grateful recipient
* feeling hurt by something someone says – let it go and B R E A T H E!

You're in the 'life is short' practice field right now! Let some things go and focus on the really important ones. You can do this – with help!

8

'AND NOW WHAT?'

'And now what?'

Tip: It is normal to feel uncertain living in an uncertain situation.

Are you:
- thinking (correctly) life is not in your control?
- feeling uncertain and anxious...?
- hearing yourself 'blithering'?

Well, what is the 'normal' response to a pressured situation like this? This is tough stuff. The news won't change just because we long for it to.

The path of caring for someone with an end-of-life diagnosis is not mapped out – even by MRIs or CAT scans. We're still left with our low-tech responses of:

'Really?'
'And now what?'
'Are you sure?'
'What matters most?'
'I love you.'
'It's not fair!'

Getting your head around something you don't want to get your head around thank-you-very-much is beyond hard. Where's the wine? (let's be real here!).

When you need support or advice, or are unsure, be willing to ask for help by:
- picking up the phone
- emailing, texting or Skyping
- inviting someone over for their opinion
- asking another person to not just advise but to take over the action

All the above are important initiatives in a pressured situation. 'Carrying on carrying on' is probably not sensible if you feel exhausted.

IT IS WHAT IT IS

When I asked medical professionals about Mike's future, there were three replies:
1. 'We don't know.'
2. 'No one knows.'
3. 'Everyone is different.'

I searched for a conversation. I was really searching for certainty . . . a map. Well, a map I liked(!).

Scans and lab tests advised the 'what' of Mike's diagnosis, and the spread of the tumours. There was no map of 'what's next'. How could there be with everyone being different and past estimates proving inaccurate?

The lack of such a map somehow kept hope alive. Oh, we saw the results of tests after the initial swirl of appointments – they weren't pretty. Treatments with an expensive 'miracle' drug gifted by a dear friend began. Then … there was mystery all around the hopeful bubble.

Accepting 'this is what it is' took months.

Caring Choices Story: Deepening uncertainty

Jackie, who cared for her husband Kevin, writes:

In my carer journey, I have gone from absolute despair to joy, as my husband Kevin (who has stage 4 melanoma and was extremely ill with 3 months to live) began a course of immunotherapy which has given him total wellness again …

If I had to say which was worse, knowing for certain that his end was near, or with him now being well but not knowing for how long, it would be a difficult choice to make. That might sound silly, because of course it is far, far better having a well husband than not – obviously I wouldn't want it any other way – but there is a part of me that just longs to know how long this reprieve is going to be.

Doctors and friends say to just enjoy the good times for as long as we have them, and of course we do, but from time to time in the back of my mind is the thought that I am probably going to have to go through the same heartbreaking grief all over again. The medical fraternity cannot/will not say how long this wonderful remission is likely to last – immunotherapy is too new, and individuals too diverse in reaction, to have any useful predictability. It could all come crashing down in a matter of months, or he could live a full lifespan with the cancer held totally at bay. We have no way of knowing, and that's hard.

Ever-watchful of his every cough, ache or pain, I know I am often paranoid, but that's the legacy of uncertainty. I do try to put the awful possibilities of the cancer resurging out of my mind, and for the most part I succeed. Just occasionally, especially when I am very tired (I haven't slept well ever since diagnosis nearly two and a half years ago), the demons come out, and I envisage life without my rock. How fortunate am I then, to have said rock to hug me, and tell me 'Hey, I'm still here, everything's going to be all right.'

Pleasance, who cared for her partner Jane, writes:

I was living with more uncertainty than I'd ever faced in my life. How long was Jane going to live? We'd been told 'a matter of months', which we'd both laughed at on leaving the hospital, and had said to each other, almost simultaneously – 'Well, that could be 12 or 24.' It felt like our private joke.

Robert, who cared for his wife Anne, writes:

I'm a practical person, so being able to administer drugs and monitor how Anne was doing helped me deal a little bit with the fact that this was something that I couldn't fix, no matter how significant it was to me, no matter how much love I expressed, no matter how much I wanted to 'make it better' ....

Caring Choices Story: Managing the transition to hospice

Pleasance, who cared for her partner Jane, writes:

When Jane needed to go into the hospice, right at the end, we realised someone would need to explain 'The Clan' to the hospice staff: we had friends that had left that night at midnight from Wellington, as soon as they'd heard Jane had been taken in. Other close friends from Auckland were already with us, around the clock, as part of this last vigil.

So, when our Wellington friends arrived, one of them, who'd also been a psychiatric nurse in a previous career, went to the nursing staff with another friend and told them about how we worked, and our concept of 'Clan' – in effect another word to describe our lesbian community. This made it a lot easier to carry on as we'd been at home – with friends around Jane and me all the way through. Giving the explanation was something I was completely incapable of doing by myself at this point. All I could think of was that Jane's death was now imminent. I was doing the best I could, to hold myself together. Friends brought food into the hospice kitchen – knowing that was definitely something I couldn't have managed! I hadn't even packed a proper bag for myself, so various friends staying at our home in Grey Lynn brought in clothes as I needed them.

9

CHOICES

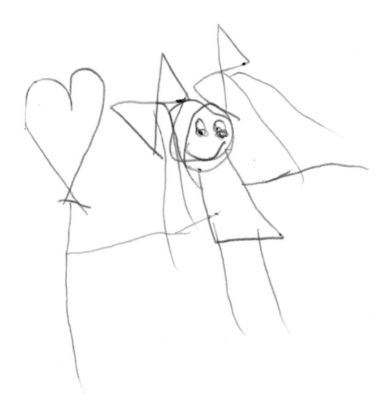

Minna's self portrait of what she called 'a love heart'.

Plateauing

Tip: A plateauing time can be an opportunity to review and plan.

'Plateauing' is my term for the common experience of chemotherapy, radiotherapy or other palliative treatments causing illness symptoms to decrease and previous activities that had no longer been possible (e.g. driving or gardening) to resume. A joyous respite from terror!

However, our previously honest conversations also plateaued amidst the joy. Plateauing is an opportunity to discuss or review priorities and preferences outlined in Section 3. I recommend that.

You can take this opportunity to think about your wishes concerning care choices too. When you are tired and the ill person fragile, it is hard to come together about subjects that are confronting. How to approach this? Read on!

Conversations that matter

Tip: This situation is likely to be new and you may not feel prepared. See what feels right to share or not to share. It is a choice.

I was anxious about 'bursting the hopeful bubble' when it was clear Mike's health was deteriorating and the joyful plateauing time had halted our honest conversations about reality… I did not have the words to revisit our honest conversations. Nor did anyone I asked. Mike remembered he was dying three days before he died and was able once more to talk honestly and lovingly with our sons and me. His dying was as gentle as his living.

Practical steps that can be taken

Tip: I know from experience that reality is not easy, my friends. I advise not to protect each other from the reality of dying until one is fragile and the other exhausted. You both know, really. A good friend of you both may assist with a heart-to-heart conversation.

The pace of physical change in people with an end-of-life illness is so varied that this page could go anywhere in this Guide. It makes sense to become familiar with end-of-life action plans because:

- at an important time of change for everyone, the more that has been thought about, discussed and planned for, the less stress and pressure there will be
- it is comforting to have plans in place with the contribution of the ill person included (if they wish to contribute) and other family members
- each family group is different and individual members of the group may have different needs and views to take into account – which takes time
- memories of this time can be long – organise for good memories!

I later learned how to begin conversations with the ill person about dying, and what is important to them, from a lecture by Dr Atul Gawande, a researcher, author and surgeon from the United States.

Dr Atul Gawande's key 'access questions' to important sharing conversations are:
- What is your understanding of where you are with your illness now?
- What are your fears and worries for the future?
- What are your goals (or main priorities) if your time is short?
- What are you willing and not willing to sacrifice (let go)?*

* Reprinted here with permission from the *New Zealand Listener* magazine, May 16–22, 2016, p. 21. The words in brackets were advised by Barbara Docherty of TADS Training.

You can redo these questions into your own words and have them in your pocket to ask the person you are caring for when the time feels right – though probably not all at once(!).

Then, simply listen. Your response at first might be companionable silence as you absorb what is said: it is a time to accept, to love and possibly to clarify what you think you heard.

Special advice to the palliative carer at home

Plan to rest while someone else is with the ill person as appropriate. Walks and sitting in the garden are examples of much-needed uninterrupted time to just be... Sensing the best next steps can become easier if we allow space. It is good to have others around us in a similar space and pace.

Conversations to have while we are well and with it*

Where would the ill person (and each of us) prefer to die? Home, hospice, hospital, elsewhere? Have this choice written down and, if at home is preferred, consider care arrangements that support both this choice and yourself as palliative carer.

* My personal opinion is that most people don't *really* think life will end – that's why so few plan for it.

Funeral director choice

Funeral directors can advise, support and guide you as a group through conversations about what happens in the end. Who will your family group choose? Please seek assistance with costs if appropriate (e.g. from Work and Income). I found our funeral director's compassionate yet matter-of-fact approach a wonderful help.

Contact and meet with a funeral director well before needed. Visit www.accidentalcarer.com for advice given by funeral director Chris Foote to ensure conversations and plans best reflect family conversations. The funeral director will advise of their services, costs and legal requirements. The choices and associated costs take time to absorb, so do plan ahead. My sister accompanied me to the funeral directors. Who might you ask beforehand to accompany you? Write down the decisions made.

Legal powers of attorney for health and property, and wills

Consult your solicitor about these or the Citizens Advice Bureau about finding local help. These can be done at any time, and are important to have in place for all of us, so why not plan ahead now? You can keep the legal Power of Attorney (property), Power of Attorney (health), and wills in one place.

If/when the GP or other medical person advises the ill person's physical changes mean they are dying, here are the choices to consider for their relevance to your situation:

- If your family member is likely to move to hospital or hospice for more care, ahead of time arrange with two people (probably members of your Home Team) for a well-supported transition as outlined by Pleasance (see page 72). This will enable you to focus on your family member and yourself while chosen others manage the ambulance, arrival at the new place, and as many of the administrative needs as they can. The particular wishes of you and the ill person learned ahead of time can be advised and taken care of. This is so supportive of exhausted and fragile people.

- If the plan is that the ill person will die at home, you and the family of the ill person may think it would be useful to have Hospice or other agency support. Hospice can recommend agencies they know provide this. It is possible to access funding for a few nights for a paid carer through some Hospices. You will need to ask.

The Advance Care Planning Guide is available at your hospital and through the Advance Care Planning website (www.advancecareplanning.org.nz) and is another way for a family group to become familiar with choices we all can make ahead of time, including medical ones.

Communication with family and friends

A group email is effective at this time. A family member may attend to this or phone calls on your behalf (they will need the contact details in advance).

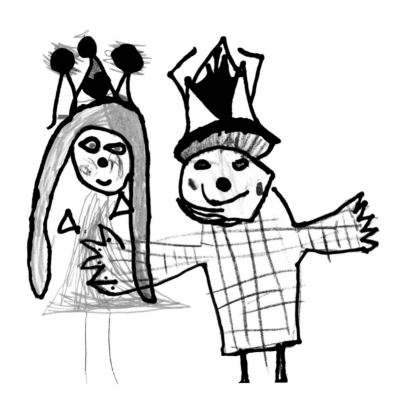

'*Princess Minna and Prince Mike*' *by Minna Capper*
Minna's beaming love helped our souls grow.

The next generation

Tip: Shall we prepare the way for them to accept dying being a natural part of living?

Sanna, the mother of our granddaughter Minna, encouraged me to involve Minna in arrangements being made for when her beloved 'Gandad' died. This was challenging territory for me but I recognised it was a healthier approach than the denial of death I had grown up with.

Minna drew pictures on a plain bed sheet of times she had enjoyed with her Gandad. After Mike died and family and friends gathered quietly around 12 hours later, Minna stood near Mike's body, touched him and used her pictures on his new bed cover to tell us all of their special times together. Fish and chips and sushi featured! I was grateful and relieved to participate in this easy introduction to our family of a healthy new tradition of death being part of life.

Minna now talks of her Gandad easily and with love.

10

SACRED MYSTERIES

Have you seen a baby born ... their eyes slowly opening, their wide-open gaze?
... a sacred transition into our world, beyond words.

Have you seen a person draw their last breath ... their eyes closed, their body still?
... a sacred transition out of our world, beyond words.

I am in wonder at the mystery of how one minute there is a spirit and the next there is not.

And with the baby, one minute their spirit is not there and the next it is.
I find being in wonder natural. I became familiar with Mystery on my three-year journey.

It *is* what it is.

What in your life is calling you?

We gathered at the Gibbs Farm Sculpture Park on the edge of the Kaipara Harbour – a place we love – to remember Mike after his death, to celebrate his life, and to grieve.

There, on a beautiful warm day in nature, a family friend read this poem by the 13th century Persian poet Rumi:

What in your life is calling you,
When all the noise is silenced,
The meetings adjourned ...
The lists laid aside,
And the Wild Iris blooms
By itself
In the dark forest ...
What still pulls on your soul?

Gifts palliative carers gained from their experiences

*'One of the outstanding "gifts" I take from that time was that I was not alone.
I only had to ask.*

*'But the most outstanding gift of all was realising that in the end love is the only
thing that matters. Everything else is wrapping paper. This has altered my frame
of reference for life.'*

– Pleasance

*'My gift was our family fully participating in a new tradition of death being part of
life, a heart warming sea-change from the past.'*

– Ros

*'The best gift for me was knowing that Anne knew I was there for her right through
until her spirit finally left.'*

– Robert

*'Illness had always frightened me. But I found that if I could focus on just one day,
and even one step, at a time, and not get caught up with anxiety over the future, I
could cope. I was amazed.'*

– Diana

*'I felt lucky and grateful to be with (Nan) when she was dying and for nothing
else to matter but her welfare … I'd give as much time as you can. Embrace the
possibility to love more than you ever thought possible.'*

– Tane

I Will Not Die An Unlived Life

I will not die an unlived life.

I will not live in fear

of falling or catching fire.

I choose to inhabit my days,

to allow my living to open me,

to make me less afraid,

more accessible;

to loosen my heart

until it becomes a wing,

a torch, a promise.

I choose to risk my significance,

to live so that which came to me as seed

goes to the next as blossom,

and that which came to me as blossom,

goes on as fruit.

DAWNA MARKOVA

Heartfelt acknowledgements

I would like to gratefully thank the home-based palliative carer contributors who were so willing to share their personal caring stories with me:

Pleasance Hansen
Jackie Holloway
Tane Tomoana
And one family wishing to remain anonymous

This guide was written with the appreciated support of the University of Auckland Te Arai Palliative Care and End of Life Research Group led by Professor Merryn Gott.

Friends, family, professional and community people giving loving practical support to this pioneering initiative and myself include:

The Capper Family: Tim, Guy, Hayley, Sanna and Minna.

Al Morrison	Les Gray
Allan Pollock	Liese Groot
Ann Smart	Lois Kay
Annie Josephson	Margaret Bedggood
Barbara Docherty	Marjorie Lewis
Baroness Sheila Hollins	Matt and Lynne Walker
Bev Silvester-Clark	Michael Fleck
Cherry Kitchingham	Murray Prior
Chris Foote	Olivier Lacoua
Christina Rogstad	Pat Gray
Devonport library	Pauline Rundle
Dr Grant Smith	Nichola Murray
Dr Martin Hollins	Raoul Ketko
Dr Nia Ellis	Robert Bell-Booth
Dr Peter Fong	Ron Sands
Dr Rex Browne	Ruth Hamilton
Dr Sally Keeling	Sabine Kalinowsky
Elisabeth Mitchell	Samantha Lacoua
Elisabeth Vaneveld	Susan Richards
Emma Gibbs	Stewart Rundle
Gillian Sheehan and the Knitting Group	The Anne Street Medical Centre
Jan Mason	The Devonport Copy Shoppe
Jenny Adlam	Toshiki Kogiso
Joan Clark	Tricia and Stewart Macpherson
John Raeburn	Trisha Joe
Julie Reger	Victoria Wigzell